COMPOUND EXERCISES- EXERCISE THE RIGHT WAY

INTRODUCTION

A compound exercise is one which targets all major muscle groups at once. It is more effective than any isolation exercise which targets only one muscle group at once. Performing compound exercises is a style of strength training which builds up muscle mass quickly, dramatically improves overall fitness while strengthening the body as a whole. Compound exercises give a boost to your power and endurance.

This book highlights 5 highly effective compound exercises. You will learn how to perform these exercise moves correctly by following the given instructions. For beginners, I have included tips to make the exercises easier, as for advanced, I will indicate to you how you can make the moves more challenging for faster results.

- Squats
- Deadlifts
- Bench press
- Pull-ups
- Lunges

We cannot deny the fact that warm-up activities should be an essential part of any exercise program and cooling down will return the body to pre-exercise conditions and reduce muscle soreness. Hence the bonus I have for you!

+ As a bonus, you get 5 WARM-UP EXERCISES and 5 COOL-DOWN STRETCHES AND EXERCISES!

SQUATS

A squat is a compound, full body exercise which means that it works muscles in your whole body. This cheap, easy-to-do-anywhere exercise proves to be highly effective if performed correctly. A squat is also a functional exercise. That is, you do squats in your everyday life without you realizing it. So, when you do squats in your fitness routine, you make it easier to perform some everyday activities which require squats such as picking up something from the floor or simply sitting on your office chair.

Benefits of Squats:

- When performing a squat, you're working multiple muscles in your body. You build and strengthen muscles in the quadriceps, hamstrings and calves. But your abs, obliques and lower back muscles also do the work.
- Squats burn more fat. More muscles burn more fat. Squats helps you pack on muscle mass and therefore helps you burn more fat. Squats also burn more calories per rep than almost any other move!
- Squats boost performance. Regularly doing your squats will help you jump higher and run faster. If you are a basketball player or an athlete, squats will help you greatly.
- Squats will challenge your posterior chain. Squats work not only the quads, but also your hamstrings and your glutes to a large extent.
- Who doesn't want the prefect, sexy looking ass anyway?

How to perform a bodyweight squat correctly?

1) Stand with feet a little wider than shoulder-width apart, hips stacked over knees and knees over ankles.

2) Roll the shoulders back and down away from the ears. Note: Allowing the back to round cause unnecessary stress on the lower back. It's important to maintain a neutral spine throughout the movement.
3) Extend arms out straight so they are parallel with the ground, palms facing down.
4) Initiate the movement by inhaling and unlocking the hips, slightly bringing them back. Keep sending hips backward as the knees begin to bend.
5) The best squats are the deepest ones your mobility allows. Optimal squat depth would be your hips sinking below the knees.
6) Engage core and, with bodyweight in the heels, explode back up to standing, driving through heels.

Beginner tips:

Try wall sits instead. The wall sit is a bit different from typical squats since you're holding a static position for a certain period of time, rather than working through an entire range of motion.
1) Stand in front of a wall (about 2 feet in front of it) and lean against it.
2) Slide down until your knees are at about 90-degree angles and hold, keeping the abs contracted, for 20-60 seconds.
3) Come back to start and repeat, holding the squat at different angles to work the lower body in different ways.

Advanced tips:

Squat using weights! You can just use your dumbbells if you are doing your squats at home or a barbell if you are at the gym. The most important part however, is to get the right form. Only shift to squatting with weights after you have mastered the correct way of squatting.

Squat with Dumbbells

1) Stand with feet hip- or shoulder-width apart.
2) Hold medium to heavy dumbbells in each hand just outside the thighs or with arms bent above the shoulders.
3) Bend the knees and lower into a squat. Stop when your knees are at 90-degree angles or before you lose the natural arch of your back.
4) At the bottom of the movement, make sure you take your hips back, as though you're about to sit in a chair. Avoid bending the knees so that they go beyond the toes.
5) Contract the glutes and legs while stabilizing your body with a strong torso.
6) Slowly stand back up without locking the knees and repeat.

Barbell Squat

1) Stand with feet hip- or shoulder-width apart.
2) Place the barbell just above the shoulders on the trapezius muscles (i.e., the 'meaty' part of the shoulders).
3) Bend the knees and lower into a squat. Stop when your knees are at 90-degree angles OR before you lose the natural arch of your back.
4) Contract the glutes and legs while stabilizing your body with a strong torso.
5) Slowly stand back up without locking the knees and repeat.

Modified versions of squats:

- ## Body-Weight Jump Squat

1) Place your fingers on the back of your head and pull your elbows back so that they're in line with your body.

2) Dip your knees in preparation to leap.
3) Explosively jump as high as you can.
4) When you land, immediately squat down and jump again.

- <u>Wide-Stance Barbell Squat</u>

1) Hold the bar across your upper back with an overhand grip.
2) Perform a squat with your feet set at twice shoulder width.

- <u>Overhead Squat</u>

1) Descend until knees and hips are fully bent or until thighs are just past parallel to floor.
2) Knees travel in direction of toes.
3) Extend knees and hips until legs are straight.
4) Return and repeat.

DEADLIFTS

A deadlift is a full-body exercise which proves to be highly effective in the sense that it is also a functional exercise. We do deadlifts in our everyday life without realising that we are actually deadlifting. From the grocery store, to moving a piece of furniture, to picking your child up off the floor, you are deadlifting. As you build solid form deadlifting in the gym, using better form when picking things up in real life will become second nature.

Benefits of a deadlift:

- Your arms, forearms, and hands hold onto the barbell and make sure the bar stays in the right position and stays stable throughout the lift.
- Your shoulders and traps hold the weight and hold it stable.
- Your back and core help keep your entire body tight and stable to help keep your spine secure.
- Your posterior chain and legs to act as a lever and lift the weight.
- It builds strength and enhance power potential to add muscle mass to the entire body.
- It develops core strength and rigidity injury prevention.

How to perform a deadlift correctly?

1) Stand with the bar above the center of your feet – your stance should be a bit more narrow than shoulder-width to give your arms room.
2) Grab the bar overhand so your arms are vertical to the floor.

3) Bend through your knees until your shins hit the bar which must remain above the middle of your feet. Shoulder-blades directly over the bar.
4) Lift your chest but don't squeeze your shoulder-blades like on Squats.
5) Just put your shoulders back & down, head in line with rest of your spine.
6) Pull - keep the bar close to your body, roll it over your knees and thighs until your hips and knees are locked. Do not lean back at the top.

Beginner tips:

- Your lift might be hampered if you are not flexible at the hips and legs. If you feel discomfort throughout the range of motion, complement your workout with some flexibility exercises.
- A good deadlift is always the result of a good setup. Period. This means that your first step in performing a deadlifting is finding proper foot and body positioning in relation to the bar or object.
- It is an essential part of the lift to hinge mainly at your hips rather than your knees and low back. What you want to do to hinge at the hips is maintain your neutral spine and push your hips back as far as you can before lowering your body to the bar.

Advanced tips:

- Pause reps - Pause reps are performed by initiating the pull and then pausing 2-4 inches off the floor for 3-5 seconds. Once the weight is held for the specified time, you will finish the movement as explosively as possible. This pause takes away the momentum gained from pulling off the floor and is great for learning how to stay tight and under control during the lift. This makes the lift much harder.

- Clusters - Cluster sets are characterized by performing heavy singles or doubles performed several times in succession but resting around ten seconds or so in between. Although this short break doesn't allow for full recovery between the mini sets, it does allow the lifter to use a weight that he or she would normally not be able to complete the desired reps without stopping.

Modified versions of deadlifts:

- ## Sumo Deadlift

1) The setup for the sumo deadlift is anywhere from slightly wider than hip width (called semi-sumo) or extremely wide with your toes almost touching the plates. Most people will fall somewhere in between these extremes.
2) It is important to make sure your toes point out – depending on the person this can be about 45 degrees to almost 90 degrees (almost straight out).
3) The grip should be directly under your shoulders. This is different than the conventional deadlift where you grab the bar outside your hips/stance.
4) As with any deadlift variation, make sure you push your hips back and down first. Unique to the sumo deadlift, your hips will start much lower than other variations and your chest higher.
5) To initiate the lift push outwards with your feet like you are trying to 'spread' the ground and give your glutes a hard squeeze.

- ## Kettlebell Deadlift

1) Make sure you start with the bell directly underneath you or in-line with your mid-foot.
2) For those with mobility restrictions, it may be better to start with a wider, sumo stance.

- Rack Pull

1) The bar height can be raised up by placing it in a power rack. This can be used to make the movement more accessible to someone who can't maintain good form when the bar on the floor or it can be used as an overload movement with heavier weight than a full deadlift.
2) If you don't have a power rack, a thick phone book or a bumper plate can be used to raise the bar to a better starting point.

BENCH PRESS

The bench press is one of the most popular exercises you'll see at a traditional gym. Once again, the bench press is a highly effective compound exercise. It targets multiple muscles at once. While there are various types of presses which all fall into the compound exercises category, bench press happens to be the most popular one due to its rather simplicity and convenience.

Benefits of a bench press:

- When the muscles at the elbow (triceps) and shoulder (deltoid) assist the chest muscles in the movement, more weight can be handled safely, and you're left with a more efficient workout.
- The simplicity of the movement can also be taken advantage of by placing your entire focus on just pushing the weight up, unlike other chest exercises that require additional balance and coordination.
- The bench press exercise activates a large number of muscle groups in the upper-half of your body. Such groups include your pecs, deltoids, your forearm muscles, hand muscles and your abdominals.

How to perform a bench press correctly?

1. Keep a tight grip on the bar at all times, a tighter grip equates to more tension in the lower arms, upper back and chest.
2. Keep your chest up (thoracic extension) throughout the movement.
3. Elbows should be tucked and end up at approximately 45 degrees from your side.

Fitness is a mental challenge not a physical one.

4. Unrack the weight and take a deep breath and hold it.
5. Row the weight down to your chest by pulling the bar apart like a bent over row. Do not relax and let the weight drop.
6. Back, hips, glutes and legs are tight and isometrically contracted.
7. When you touch your chest, drive your feet downward and reverse the movement.
8. Lock out the elbows without losing your arch and thoracic extension.

Beginner tips:

- Weight Acclimation - Incrementally build your way up to the heavier weights that you'll be using during the bench press. Your body and your mind must be prepped for lifting heavy loads. So, stay on the safe side and start with weights which you can handle very well at first.
- You absolutely have to make sure you have the right technique before starting this exercise! Practice with light dumbbells or no weights. Pretend like you are actually lifting off a heavy barbell and do the exact same thing you would do. This will allow you to build up the form and avoid injury later on.
- Strengthen Opposing Muscles. One of the most effective, yet overlooked bench press tips is to improve your strength on **back exercises** and **bicep exercises**. The back and biceps are the major opposing muscle groups involved in this exercise. The stronger these muscles are, the more potential you have for adding weight to the bench press and developing the muscles involved in the movement.

Advanced tips:

Decline Bench Press

One of the best things about the decline bench press is that you can use a bit more weight on it than you can on the regular flat bench due to the change in biomechanics and somewhat decreased range of motion.

1. Set up a bench press station by adjusting a bench to a 45-degree decline or use a decline bench station.
2. Grasp the bar with an overhand grip, hands about shoulder-width apart.
3. Hook the tops of your feet under the pads at the end of the bench.
4. Lift the bar off the rack and lower it down to chest level in a smooth and controlled motion.
5. Push the bar straight up, resisting the tendency for the bar to move backwards due to the decline.

Modified versions of Bench Press:

- Floor Press - With reduced range of motion, your chest muscles will not fully activate, leaving most of the work to your triceps.

1. Lie on your back on a mat in the middle of a free weight rack with your knees bent and your feet flat on the floor.
2. Adjust the height of the bar to where you usually perform a Bench Press.
3. Grasp the bar with an overhand grip, hands about shoulder-width apart.
4. Lift the bar off the rack and then lower it in a smooth and controlled motion until your triceps touch the ground.
5. Push the bar straight up, keeping your knees bent and feet flat on the floor.

- <u>Close-Grip Bench Press</u> - This variation also focuses on building the triceps. Grasp the bar with your hands close together. Just like with the Floor Press, your chest muscles are not fully activated, requiring your triceps to work harder.

1. Set up a bench press station with a flat bench.
2. Grasp the bar with an overhand grip, hands close together.
3. Lift the bar off the rack and lower it in a smooth and controlled motion until the bar almost touches your chest.
4. Push the bar straight up while trying to keep the bar level.

PULL-UPS

Pull-ups force you to lift your own body-weight. They are the best strength training exercises you can do for upper-body strength & muscle mass. Unfortunately Pull-ups are hard. However, they are also a fundamental upper-body compound exercise. The effort will definitely be worth the pain.

Benefits of a pull-up:

- Pull-ups are very convenient to perform. They can be done with nothing more than a pull-up bar. If you do not have access to one, you can also use an open beam, the edge of a deck or you can visit a local park and use a set of monkey bars. This makes it possible to build strength with limited equipment.
- Grip Strength - Pull-ups can help develop powerful forearms and grip strength to help improve your performance in several sports. Activities like martial arts and wrestling require a strong grip.
- You can boost the intensity of your back workout simply by strapping a weight plate to your waist or hanging a kettlebell from your foot while you perform your pullups.
- Pull-ups will get your heart rate up and really kick your butt. If you want to boost the fat loss capabilities of doing pull-ups you could decrease the time in between sets and also super set your pull-ups with another exercise.

How to perform a pull-up correctly?

1. Grasp the bar with hands outside shoulder width and palms facing away from you.

2. Use your legs to jump into the top position of the pull-up, so your chin is over the bar.
3. From there, slowly lower your body down to a dead hang.
4. Try to make it last five seconds.

Beginner tips:

- If you really find yourself struggling with a single pull-up, try a chin-up until you make your way through to a pull-up. The difference is that during Pull-ups, your palms face away which means less biceps and more back. During chin-ups, your palms face you which mean your biceps work more. Chin-ups are easier than pull-ups.
- Ask For Help. Ask someone to grab your side with his hands. Let him help you on the way up by squatting down & pressing up.

Advanced tips:

- Weighted Pull-Up

There are three primary ways to add weight:
1. Use a weight.
2. Put a dumbbell in between your ankles when crossed or use an ankle weight.
3. Use a weighted vest.

Modified versions of Bench Press:

- Muscle-Ups

1) Lift your entire torso over the bar so that it's high enough to then extend your arms straight.

2) Keep your legs slightly forward as you are coming down (20 degree angle).
3) Swing them backwards to help you forcefully pull up.

- ## L-Sit Pull Up

1) Hang from a pull-up bar.
2) With your legs straight, bend at the waist and bring your legs up 90 degrees, making sure not to lean backward.
3) Once your legs are up, perform a Pull-Up while maintaining the "L" shape throughout the motion.

- ## Side-to-Side Pull-Up

1) Perform a standard Pull-Up.
2) After your head clears the bar, flex the biceps of one arm so your body and head move laterally toward that arm.
3) Flex the other arm and perform the same movement.
4) Lower yourself. That's one rep.

LUNGES

The lunge exercise is one of the best exercises that you can do for your thighs and glutes. It's a great exercise that can be performed anywhere. The lunge can be a difficult exercise to master. However if you get the technique right, it's an effective exercise that can be performed with or without exercise equipment. Lunges also target multiple muscle groups at once.

Benefits of lunges:

- Lunges improve whole-body control, which is essential to protecting the spine during walking, running, or stair-climbing. Being a functional exercise, a lunge improves your everyday activities in many ways.
- Lunges strengthen your buttocks and legs. Strengthening these large muscle groups can speed up your metabolism, which is beneficial if you're trying to lose weight. When excess fat is reduced from your lower body, lunges can help you shape, tone and firm up your tush and legs.
- Lunges can improve your core strength. When doing lunges, you must engage your core muscles, including your back and abdominals, to keep your body upright and balanced as you move your hips up and down.

How to perform a basic lunge correctly?

1) Stand with your feet together, keep your head up and your shoulders back, place your hands on your hips and as you are facing forward choose a place to keep your eyes focused on as your perform the exercise.
2) Take a big lunge forward with your first leg and your forward leg should be bent at about a 90 degree angle.

3) Your thigh should be parallel with the ground and your back knee should be nearly touching the ground, your back leg should also be bent at a 90 degree angle.
4) Keep your body as controlled and still as possible.
5) Use your front leg to push yourself back up, push off with your front heel until you're standing straight up with your feet together.
6) Repeat with your other leg.

Beginner tips:

- Master the technique using your body weight only before attempting this exercise, especially if you have never performed the lunge before. Only add weights once you are completely at ease with doing lunges correctly.

Advanced tips:

1) Set up to do a basic lunge, but this time step your right foot out on a diagonal, not straight ahead, as if the foot is pointing to 2 o'clock on a clock face. (When you lunge with the left foot, step it out to 10 o'clock.)
2) The change in foot placement makes it harder to balance.
3) As you get stronger, try it with your hands interlaced behind your head or hold a dumbbell in each hand to increase resistance.

Modified versions of Lunges:

- Walking lunges

1) Stand with your shoulders in neutral posture and draw in your core.

2) Step forward, gliding your foot along the ground until your heel touches a few feet in front of you.
3) As your front toe lands, bend your front and rear legs, lowering down until your rear knee is about 1 inch above the floor.
4) Your front heel should be directly below your knee.
5) Both legs should be bent at around a 90 degree angle.
6) From the bottom position you have many options. For the basic lunge, lift your body up at the same time you bring your hips and rear foot forward until you are in the original standing position.

- ## Karate Kick Backs

1) Begin in a traditional lunge position with left foot forward, both knees slightly bent, and hands firmly on hips.
2) Lower body, dropping right knee until it is approximately one inch from the floor.
3) Kick right heel up to glute.
4) Lower back into a lunge and repeat.
5) Keep your chin parallel to the floor throughout the entire move to avoid bending too far forward at the hip when you are kicking.

- ## Lunges with Lateral Raises

1) Stand up with a pair of dumbbells held at your sides. Your upright upper body posture should remain constant for the duration of your lunges.
2) Draw in your core as you take a deep breath.
3) Lunge one foot forward, gliding it along a couple inches above the floor.
4) Land on your heel and set your toes down while keeping the majority of your weight on your heel.

5) Lower your body toward the ground.
6) As your back knee approaches the floor, pause with your torso upright in the middle of both legs which should be at congruent 90 degree angles.
7) Perform a lateral raise and lower your arms as you lunge back up to the original position.

- ## Lunges with Biceps Curls and Shoulder Press

1) Get focused and stand up tall with a pair of dumbbells at your side. Keep your core tight and your upper body should be upright for the duration of this entire complex movement.
2) Lunge forward as usual putting your heel down first and making sure your upper body is in the center of gravity.
3) Perform a biceps curl when your body is completely stable at the bottom of the lunge.
4) After you perform your curl keep the dumbbells at shoulder level in a high-hang position.
5) Lunge back up to a balance and perform a shoulder press.
6) Try to keep your balance and let the weights come all the way down to your sides at the original position and repeat.

5 WARM-UP EXERCISES

Warm-up activities should be an essential part of any exercise program. The purpose of warming up is to prepare the body for the conditioning or stimulus of the exercise session by increasing blood flow to the heart and to the exercising muscles, which serves to warm up and loosen up muscles.

A dynamic warm-up uses stretches that are "dynamic," meaning you are moving as you stretch. Dynamic stretching is ideal as the core of a warm-up routine for several reasons:

1. It activates muscles you will use during your workout.
2. Dynamic stretching improves range of motion.
3. Dynamic stretches improve body awareness.
4. Warming up in motion enhances muscular performance and power.

Below are 5 exercises which you use in your warm-up routine:

1) High Kicks

- If starting with your right leg, extend your left arm straight out.
- Kick your leg up while keeping your leg and hand straight so that your toes hit your palm.
- Try to progressively kick higher, but complete this exercise while staying under control.

2) Jump Squats

- Stand up with your feet about shoulder width apart while holding your hands behind your head, or on your hips.
- Squat down until the hips are about parallel with the ground.
- Forcibly jump off the ground.
- Land softly and repeat the jump.

3) Sideways Shuffle

- With your legs wide apart and toes pointed forward, side lunge to the left.
- Shift weight to the right side for another lunge.
- Follow with two shuffles to the left, stopping in a lunge to the left to repeat the sequence again.
- Go one direction for 10 reps, and then switch sides.

4) Standing Lunges With Dumbbells

- Stand with your torso upright holding two dumbbells in your hands by your sides. This will be your starting position.
- Step forward with your right leg around 2 feet or so from the foot being left stationary behind and lower your upper body down, while keeping the torso upright and maintaining balance.
- Inhale as you go down. Note: As in the other exercises, do not allow your knee to go forward beyond your toes as you come down, as this will put undue stress on the knee joint. Make sure that you keep your front shin perpendicular to the ground.
- Using mainly the heel of your foot, push up and go back to the starting position as you exhale.
- Repeat the movement with the left leg.

5) Stork Fly

- Stand with feet together and extend arms to shoulder height, palms facing up.
- Raise left knee so thigh is almost parallel to floor. Keep hips level. Hold for 10 to 15 seconds.
- With left knee lifted, bend torso forward, extend left leg back, and raise arms overhead until arms, torso, and left leg are parallel to floor.
- Hold for 10 to 15 seconds, and then slowly return to start.
- Switch legs and repeat.

BONUS!

5 COOL-DOWN STRETCHES AND EXERCISES

Cooling down will return the body to pre-exercise conditions and reduce muscle soreness. Take the time to lower your heart rate through about five minutes, and then perform stretches. Stretching improves flexibility, helps to disperse lactic acid that can build up during the exercise session and helps to prepare the body for the next workout.

Below are 5 exercises which you use in your cool-down routine:

1) Inner Thigh Stretch

- For the inner thigh stretch, sit down with your back straight and bend your legs, putting the soles of your feet together.
- Holding on to your feet, try to lower your knees towards the floor.

2) Hamstring Stretch

- To do a hamstring stretch, lie on your back and raise your right leg.
- Keeping your left leg bent with your foot on the floor, pull your right leg towards you keeping it straight.
- Don't hold at the knee level.
- Repeat with opposite leg.

3) Calf Stretch

- For the calf stretch, step your right leg forward, keeping it bent and lean forwards slightly.
- Keep your left leg straight and try to lower the left heel to the ground.
- Repeat with opposite leg.

4) Side stretch

- Place your feet hip width apart.
- Slowly slide your right hand down your right leg.
- You should feel a slight stretch down the left hand side of your body.
- Return to the starting position and repeat to the left.

5) Quadriceps stretch

- Sit on the edge of a chair.
- Bend the leg underneath your seat and rest your toes on the floor
- Hold.
- Repeat with the other leg.

For more information on health and fitness, visit my blog at
http://yourfitnesshealth.blogspot.com/

Do not forget to subscribe for latest updates!

You can also find my facebook page at
https://www.facebook.com/yourfitnesshealthblog

Follow for latest updates!

www.ingramcontent.com/pod-product-compliance
Lightning Source LLC
Chambersburg PA
CBHW050803290526
45792CB00008B/2306